Valley to Victory

Andrea J. Riley

©Copyright 2021 Andrea J. Riley

All rights reserved. This book is protected under the copyright laws of the United States of America.

ISBN-13: 978-1-7361198-8-4

No portion of this book may be reproduced, distributed, or transmitted in any form, including photocopying, recording, or other electronic or mechanical methods, without the written permission of the publisher, except in the case of brief quotations embodied in reviews and certain other non-commercial uses permitted by copyright law. Permission granted on request.

For information regarding special discounts for bulk purchases, please contact LaBoo Publishing Enterprise at staff@laboopublishing.com

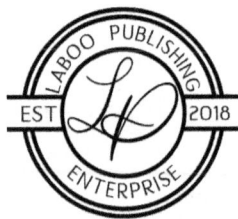

Scripture quotations marked (NIV) are taken from the Holy Bible, New International Version®, NIV®. Copyright © 1973, 1978, 1984, 2011 by Biblica, Inc.™ Used by permission of Zondervan. All rights reserved worldwide. www.zondervan.com

The Holy Bible, King James Version. Cambridge Edition: 1769; King James Bible Online, 2019. www.kingjamesbibleonline.org.

Acknowledgements

Thank you, God, for allowing the valleys that have turned to testimony that I may be able to share and encourage others. Thank you for blessing me to be a mother to three wonderful children to share my journey through life with. Thank you to my family and those who are referenced in this journey and those who are not referenced (in this one) who have either unknowingly or knowingly sown seeds in my life along this journey. Lord, I don't take it lightly to have been chosen for this assignment.

Table of Contents

Introduction 1

Chapter 1: Girl, you are a hot mess! 3

Chapter 2: What is this twitching?
Am I having a stroke? 9

Chapter 3: The transformation process 13

Chapter 4: Freedom from Bondage 17

Chapter 5: Learning to let my flesh die daily 23

Chapter 6: Come out swinging and unashamed 27

Chapter 7: Learning to walk 33

Chapter 8: Whew, all this comes with being Saved? . . . 37

Chapter 9: Leaving the Broken, Bitter Girl
in the Last Decade 39

Chapter 10: Freedom from Church Hurt 41

Chapter 11: How hard is Godly Discipline? 45

Chapter 12: The day I decided to stop robbing God! 47

Chapter 13: Lord, I just got off the Walker; how am I going to show someone how to use it? . . . 51

Chapter 14: The journey continues; PRESS FORWARD 57

Afterword 59

Introduction

I used to wonder why me? Lord, what are the chances one person could endure so much heartache in a lifetime? Why the molestation, rape, abuse, brokenness, depression, hard times and suffering?

It was necessary, and for such a time as THIS! To be able to be a light to show that in God you have VICTORY! Regardless of what it looks like, we have already won!

It is my prayer that my testimony resonates in your spirit so brightly that you are able to WALK into a more loving, powerful and anointed life with the Father.

Love,

Chapter 1
Girl, you are a hot mess!

When you look at me what do you see?

She has been broken. She has covered herself with fig leaves to hide the pain of molestation, date rape, abusive relationships, dismay, depression and suicide attempts. She has been abused, angry and bitter. While a teenager she has carried two babies that did not survive, not knowing how to even handle such pain. She has cried many tears. She has stood in hospital rooms and held hands, watching last breaths of people she thought she couldn't live without. She has been without and no one knew. She has been unable to get out of bed because she was in such a dark place. She has used food, drugs and alcohol to numb the pain when no one was watching. She has been in relationships with other women. She has been a mother who was so depressed she contemplated suicide and taking her kids with her. She has been unable to find joy in the face of her children even though she desperately wanted to.

NEVERTHELESS, she is blessed. Through all the storms, God kept her on a steady path to right now. She is a mother with a successful public sector career. She is an Airman serving her country. She is a college graduate with Bachelor's, Master's and Doctoral-level Education Specialist degrees. She is a travel agent. She has sat on boards, managed nonprofits and even coordinated events, both professional and personal. She is covered by grace in the place of fig leaves now. She is free from the bondage that held her captive far too long. She is breaking out of the generational curses that bind her families and is attempting to bring them with her. One of those women she dated became one of her best earthly friends and supporters in life and their relationship went from romance to sisterhood. She has surrendered to God and watched him move on her behalf. She is not perfect but she is a work in progress and is literally a living testimony!

She is me and I am her.

The reality is that right now, at the turn of a decade, I am learning to Walk: Walking in Faith, Walking in Love, Walking in Peace, Walking in Freedom, and Walking in Deliverance. The undeniable crippling of life can blindly disable our ability to Walk. We wake up each day with our feet hitting the ground so we walk in the physical yet are incapacitated in the spiritual, emotional, and mental. We sometimes go through life in a bit of a fog. That is ok. When we walk through fog and it clears, we are in awe at the ability to see again. As people, we can work and live while battling pain and depression, and sometimes even while actively planning our suicide. Yet we are smiling and laughing as the INSIDE of us is dying! This place of disability can hinder our God-given destiny. It can disable the Faith we attempt to Walk in each day.

The journey from being Disabled to Walking is one of Faith, Depression, Tears, Restoration and DELIVERANCE.

Ten years ago God told me I would write a book. I started but I couldn't finish it. Five years ago, God put the book back on my heart. I still didn't move. Now here I sit after praying on this BOOM moment in my journey to deliverance and freedom in Christ. I sat writing and compiling my journey! I said, "Lord, I can't write a book." He said to me, "It is already written; go back to your social media, phone notes, and handwritten entries. There is the journey I want you to share." Before I would have been writing in pain, not helping anyone, probably damaging people trying to help them while I was still in a valley and damaged myself. Now I write from PEACE and DELIVERANCE, WHILE WALKING!

After January 2014, I stayed off social media for over a year because I couldn't handle the death of my high school sweetheart. I blocked anyone connected with him so I wouldn't see their posts. I got back on to be present and to engage but rarely posted. I just shared and commented. In 2018 I began to post more, broken and trying to be positive but still broken! At certain points from 2014 to 2018, I would ghost social media and not even have access to it on purpose. I closed myself off from family, with only limited and very brief interactions. I was hurting in ways no one but God could understand and heal. I realized I needed time to grieve and get MYSELF together so I decided not to date or enter a relationship until God got me to a place where I felt I was ready. If you knew me and my high school sweetheart's relationship and friendship, until he gained his wings, you would know I didn't need to take the hurt, anger, and bitterness from his death into another relationship and create toxicity because no man could ever fill that void in my mind and heart during that time. Relationship or not.

I learned more about me during that time than I had in all my years of living.

In 2017, I began attending a small group called Freedom. Because of the time, I was unable to fully commit and attend like I wanted and needed to. Yet I was never the same. I was still in a very dark place, suicidal and even homicidal at times. It was horrible to be there and I knew God would bring me out, but I sure was praying for him to hurry up. I went through the same small group again in 2020, and what a freeing experience it was.

In 2018, as I attempted to reenter the dating world for the first time since 2014, I was date raped. When the enemy couldn't use my childhood trauma anymore, he started throwing darts in adulthood. The Monday after it happened, I was on my way out the door to work and something took hold of me. I called my little sister and told her to come cut all this hair off my head. When she made it over that morning, I was a complete mess. She was trying to figure out what in the world my problem was. I told her what happened and she said, "For women hair is something we control, and you feel like he took a sense of control from you. You're gonna be ok." My mama reverted ALL the way back to before she was saved, saying, "Invite him over for Thanksgiving dinner so I can get your uncles and brothers to beat the hell out him." While the offer was tempting, I declined. The therapist said, "When you are walking out of the emotional bondage of the trauma you will want hair again. You will be able to tolerate hair again."

When it happened, even though emotionally I was broken, spiritually I was praying, "Lord, I don't want to hate him. Lord, just get me through it."

I knew from my misery and torment from my childhood trauma that I didn't want hate on the inside of me anymore. I didn't want despair and bitterness inside me. I enrolled in counseling for about six months to help me work through the process.

In 2018, my feet began to tingle. I was invited to the church I knew to attend. I walked in not knowing what to expect, but I knew what I needed. I grew up heavily in the church but baby, I was lost, wandering in the wilderness. During this time I was sexually assaulted by a guy I was getting to know. I was re-traumatized from being molested as a child. I felt I was spiraling again but I kept making sure to pay attention to the tingling. Instead of focusing on him and the rape, I kept my eyes on God. That was a familiar place that I knew I didn't like. I knew I needed help and I intentionally sought it out. While I knew from growing up in the church that God had me, common sense said, GIRL GET SOME HELP!

Chapter 2
What is this twitching? Am I having a stroke?

In 2019, the tingle turned into a twitching. From January to August I was still just twitching. I knew I was waking up but I was just twitching. God was manifesting in ways unimaginable despite the storms, struggles, sickness and death wreaking havoc in my family. Be careful what you ask God for. I had been battling with taking the "Walk" I knew to be in my life for years. Intentionally surrendering more and more in 2018-2019, I shifted to saying, "Lord I am ready to do this. I am open to do this but God I don't know how to move these feet!" When I tell you in two days I met, heard & witnessed more anointed, powerful women of god than I have in my whole 33 years on this earth, I am talking about the real ones. Not the ones who go to church on Sunday then tear down the people they hug on Sunday morning. Not the ones who really don't even look at the Bible except Sunday when they get dressed up to walk in the House to really spectate. Not the ones who say AMEN but really don't even know how to draw people through the love of God because they are too busy condemning them because they think they are perfect. Not the ones who are more concerned about their Sunday best than about not only your soul but their own.

God will place you in an anointed atmosphere to show you just how to Walk! He will put a mirror in front of you to show you "this is what I've been trying to get you to see. This is what I've been trying to save you for! This moment at this place is what I needed you to know so when the enemy tries to tell you that you can't be called, you can't be anointed, you can't minister to people, you can tell the enemy I know a team of women—and men, for that matter—who walk this walk every day and if you don't back up, we're gonna walk all over you, devil."

I remember all the things in my life that could have taken me out but God protected me. I now understand when Pastor Young used to preach and he would reference Jeremiah 20:9 and say, "It is like fire shut up in my bones" when I can't hold it any longer!

Then it happened! November 2019, I began to move my feet one at a time, kind of like therapy, slow and steady, just raising them. Like a baby, I was grabbing the Word of God in my life that was gonna help me move my feet but would help me hold steady. I began to pull up and walk around things that stood between me, God and his purpose for my life, still holding on because I was afraid to fall.

I started taking notes on my phone and sharing them from lessons taught on Sundays and that I listen to while working out each day. It helped me begin to study with a different mindset, not just rereading notes but researching different translations and all that. Key words began to jump out at me. I began to study harder in God's word than ever before. I wanted such a relationship with him that no one could take it away, not even the enemy. I wanted, when those dark days hit, to be able to stand in that authority and command the enemy to move.

This Journey of my mental and spiritual transformation process still amazes me. It still is so hard for me to fathom how awesome God is in his grace and mercy. It was one Sunday as my Pastor, Gregg Magee Sr., pointed out how I had begun to use my social media platform for accountability by posting my workouts and studies from the Word that I realized that while my intention in posting was solely to share the journey so someone knew they were not alone, in a sense he was certainly correct. The accountability was not hinged on what people thought of me personally but more so they could see the growth. The ironic part is while doing this, I knew I was changing but until I went back and reflected on my social media posts, I didn't realize just how much God had significantly transformed me mentally and spiritually by granting me the ability to do so physically.

On December 31, 2019 as I sat in church weeping and smiling, the last speaker of the night said, "I was crying from a place of strength." This wiped away any doubt, any second guessing I thought I had at the wonderful place I was in. I realized I was not weeping because I was sad, upset or bound but I wept because I was joyous, thankful and in a place of peace. I had never known that place but now I was there and I was overwhelmed with emotion.

I was finally allowing God to be the head and his Word to penetrate the depths of my soul.

As you read further, you will see excerpts from notes, written prayers and social media posts throughout the year that helped me see my own journey and growth. Some struggles and storms briefly shared will eventually flourish into a book when God moves me to do so.

It is my prayer that in reading this, you find that you too can begin to **WALK** by noticing the tingle, twitching, grasping, struggling to remain steady and finally **WALKING**. I pray that the Words you read, like the Words I heard from various people noted in this book and the Words I read, will resonate and awaken the spirit of God in the very depths of your soul.

Chapter 3
The transformation process

What a year 2019 was. I was in no way spiritually, emotionally or mentally prepared for the transformation my life was about to take! As I reflected on social media I began to see the changes that others told me they saw in me.

January 1, 2019

It has been a long Journey. God has always blessed me to be able to talk to anyone, openly share and often inspire those around me. After months of work, we are finally at this point. The hardest part has been being quiet!

January 17, 2019
The day I learned the difference between being rich and being wealthy.

"Rich talks softly, Wealth Whispers, Broke Screams!" – Bishop Joseph Walker III.

That means people on social media "Balling" really are broke. So stop trying to be like people you think are balling. Learn what real Wealth is. People who are wealthy in reality don't care to waste money on things to impress others. They are too busy building!! Stop trying to look wealthy and build real Wealth.

That's Dripping! Now, don't comment misquoting the word. Let me go ahead and say it. 1 Timothy 6:10 states, "For the love of money is the root of all evil: which while some coveted after, they have erred from the faith, and pierced themselves through with many sorrows." NOT MONEY IS the root of all evil. It is the Love of the money that brings forth the sin.

January 19, 2019

If you are mentally, emotionally and spiritually in the same place you were five or ten years ago…… rethink your choices. Growth is action and sometimes outgrowing people, habits and choices can propel us into places we never thought imaginable. I made the choice years ago to not surround myself with people, even family, who don't share common interests. That is not being bougie or uppity; that is being grown and mature. For a person to think the choice of an adult not to partake of or participate in things they have interest in or among people they don't want to be around is bougie or uppity that, my friends, speaks volumes about your immature mindset.

Matthew 10:14 KJV – And whosoever shall not receive you, nor hear your words, when ye depart out of that house or city, shake off the dust from your feet.

Chapter 3

That means move on.

Feb. 20, 2019
I realized that "religion" and being "religious" don't mean you are saved.

I am sick and tired of people condemning others. There is a difference between condemning someone and holding them accountable. As Christians we are to hold one another accountable. But ask yourself, where is it coming from? Are you doing it out of genuine love and concern for that person? Or are you simply condemning them because YOU don't like what they do? Be careful in your journey of using the Word, religion and traditional perceptions to condemn people. In many cases, we are raised to think if we are saved or if we get saved, nothing bad happens to us. I BEG TO DIFFER!

Chapter 4
Freedom from Bondage

People don't understand the grip bondage has on us. Many of us have been bound by things in our own hearts. This was a hard concept for me to understand. How am I holding myself bound because they offended me? I had to pick that stretcher up and walk to gain release.

We carry bondage from childhood, adulthood, family ties, etc. and wonder why we are going in circles. It is tough to be released from the things that hold us in bondage, BUT when we decide we no longer want to be bound, the work BEGINS!

It is not easy to start the journey to freedom and being saved, and it sure isn't easy all the time not to let those binding chains wrap around you again.

I'm not lying back down on that stretcher. Regardless of how hard I have to claw my way out repeatedly, I still refuse to go backwards.

March 4, 2019–The day I decided I was walking out of the bondage of anger because of an absent biological father.

I have never been one to force myself in anyone's life, not even family. However, I have always wanted to make sure everyone is included, especially in family stuff. Now, I don't care. Stay bitter, angry and whatever other emotions you have about whatever it is. I am tired of dealing with all these adults, most of them older than me, who have all these issues with absent parents, siblings, etc. and always want to project that negative mess on others. You are welcome to feel however, just do it away from me. You want to let that hate and bitterness take you to hell, go ahead. Get counseling, sit on somebody's couch. Stop blaming the other person because much of the reason your life is where it is, is due to your choices! Talk to that person or don't talk to them but don't spread your bitterness to everyone then wonder why no one wants to invite you to stuff or include you. Most of the time when people take time to actually talk things out, they find things are not always how they perceive them.

My daddy was absent, unengaged and antisocial and he lived in my grandparents' back yard. Guess what? That's still my daddy and I'm still going to see about him. Regardless of what he didn't do, I will always be the best daughter I can to him.

March 5, 2019—The day I walked out of the shame of having bariatric surgery. I prayed before having the surgery that God would let my journey be about the whole me not just the physical health. Boy, did He show up and show out!

Chapter 4

No surgery is a quick fix. It takes a lot of work and discipline to maintain the weight loss over time. On February 21, 2019 I was wheeled into surgery to get the gastric sleeve. Surgery went well; weight loss has been even better. I realized how addicted to food I was. How I depended on food to fill a void or make things better when I was stressed out. During the transformation process, the stripping away of many things not of God (I prayed for this), my food and dependency on food was probably one of the hardest. I have struggled with severe obesity preventing me from passing my PT test for over five years and at times I was incapable of even doing one due to the medical illness associated with my overweight body. I asked God to help me in a way that I couldn't deny it was him, to give me the tools needed to not only do it but also maintain it day after day, using my physical health journey to draw me closer and closer to him. Let me tell you, He completely showed out this past almost two years. I have been speechless, overcome with joy and praise and even just completely blown away by what God has manifested in my life in this season.

I had been struggling one week with some food (my drug) because even though I can't eat more than three ounces I have had to refocus my attention to cut certain things back out of my lifestyle. I had been praying, asking God to give me something to help me. Some people need help. Food can be an addiction. Before judging someone, educate yourself. Bariatric surgeries are not easy ways out. They don't fix the issue, they help it—kind of like a nicotine patch for a person who is trying to quit smoking. While you drink, some eat. While you smoke weed or do other drugs, some eat. While you jump from one bed to another, some eat. In a culture where food is taught to be a comfort, many of us grow up and we want food to comfort us when we are sad, mad, angry, stressed and even happy.

I kept restating, "Obedience is better than sacrifice."

So I said, "Let me see what Bishop Joseph Walker III preached about last night." BOOM.

"Peace is not the absence of tension and trouble; it is the revelation of God's presence in your life" – Bishop Joseph Walker III

March 10, 2019–The day I reconciled with my younger cousin/daughter after a nasty falling out. While I knew I hadn't personally done anything to wrong her, I had to learn that people deal with pain differently and I knew where her pain stemmed from even if she didn't realize it.

When my uncle and aunt passed I knew NOTHING about parenting a child in high school. I was 20 or 21 years old. All I knew was she needed to finish and go to college. I thank God for blindly leading us to help one another grow. While it killed me to cut ties for four years, it was necessary for our growth as adults. She knows and understands when I need space and respects that. Now, she still acts like the spoiled teenager she was back then; she's the only person who can come home to visit and MAKE me cook what she wants. The ironic part is I had never really sat down to think how her parents' deaths affected her because like me, she has always been "the strong one." I knew it affected her in some form but I never really stopped to think how it took an emotional

Chapter 4

and mental toll on her and made her feel like she had to step in and be the mother even though she was a middle child. I had to get out of my feelings and do what I had promised my uncle, and that was to always make sure I saw about his kids. No matter how much she got on my nerves, I made a promise.

Chapter 5

Learning to let my flesh die daily

It was March 16, 2019, a few days after we found out my dad had stage 4 cancer. I prayed for God's will to be done and not to let him suffer long if he wanted to give him rest. He was officially diagnosed March 19, 2019 and gained his wings June 25, 2019. During the time he was ill, some family members were spreading news of his condition secondhand when they hadn't even called or come to see him. Their information was false and it angered me because people will post on social media and call the church folk as if they are genuinely concerned when in reality they don't care one way or the other. My father's death taught me a lot about people–specifically, how people who proclaim to be saved can be truly lost in a wilderness of religion and legalism, but that is a book for another day.

April 27, 2019 – The day we had to face the passing of my great-aunt, who had filled the void of being all the older cousins' mother, grandmother and great-grandmother in this last decade. In my depressive state I had purposely distanced myself from my family. I

would get angry when I was around them; I didn't want to stay around them long. It was nothing they did personally but just various memories, and anger because people were dying. It was depressing and made me anxious.

As we went into that week, I couldn't help but love and laugh at my crazy Roberts family! We may not always see eye to eye but we are always there for one another. We laugh together, cry together and will fight together! We have the famous 11 to thank for the love and bond we have. We know it will hurt forever but we also watched the strength of the seven brothers and sisters who are now gone as they endured everything the world threw at them and kept pushing, just like the four were left at that time. You can call the Roberts a lot of things BUT the one thing you can never say is that we don't love one another!

May 29, 2019 – The day I began to stop allowing others' chaos to determine my peace.

Refusing to allow someone who you have experienced chaos with into your everyday life or circle of peace does not mean you do not like them; it means you've learned who they were before and you know better than to allow them in that space to do so again.

There is a difference and some people should learn that. Just because you forgive people does not mean you have to befriend them. With growth comes maturity. As an adult, I make the choice if I want to speak, hold a conversation or even deal with someone. If I choose not to, THAT IS MY CHOICE. It doesn't necessarily come from a bad place, it is just my choice.

Chapter 5

Even before I became an adult, I did not surround myself with a lot of people and had a select few that I dealt with. As an adult, that number is even smaller.

May 29, 2019 – The day I realized that my parents were actually aging. The moment I saw that no matter how much I wanted to keep them on this earth, one day God would call them home.

As children, our parents and grandparents care for us entirely; as adults the roles reverse. Often we care for them even to the point of bathing and dressing them if needed. While it is not ideal, there is a blessing. They get to see the love and care they poured into you physically given back to them.

I can't wait to say, "Girl, tell yo' mama to come here and help me get this dress on and give me my teeth out that bathroom" when I'm about 90 years old and dare Kamari to blink an eye when she gets in there.

June 29, 2019 – The day I figured out that obedience is better than sacrifice. I had been keeping my eye on God, trying to draw closer while my dad was leaving us. It hurt. I was in unimaginable pain. Even after praising God he didn't suffer long, my flesh was still in pain. Even lying in bed with him, thanking God for his life, thanking him for being such a great father, my flesh was screaming, "I want my dad back."

As I cleaned my parents' room four days after my father took his last breath in that very room, in that very bed, my heart just ached. I missed Daddy so bad and wasn't sure how to go forward without him here with us. Losing a parent leaves an unimaginable void. I felt I was pretty strong and I knew beyond a shadow of a doubt that God had us through it all, yet the pain still lingered.

From June 2019 I continued to share my journey in life and on social media with one purpose: Someone will see my journey and know that with God ALL things are possible.

It was December 1, 2019 and the year had truly been a year of transformation for me and my household. I had to learn so much about myself physically, spiritually, emotionally and mentally. I had to face harsh realities over and over that year. I had to really dig deep and surrender to God, even though I was half-surrendering all my life. In 2020 I was ready to continue my growth and help others continue to grow.

I had to learn to love myself all over again and remove emotional baggage that was keeping me bound.

Chapter 6
Come out swinging and unashamed

November 29, 2019 – When I shredded Religion and Legalism, understanding that God's love is not conditional based on a religion or denomination.

Please stop telling people if they're not trying to live right, ain't no point in them going to church! THAT IS THE PLACE THEY NEED TO BE TO HELP THEM IN LIFE, REGARDLESS OF HOW THEY LIVE. That is the most ignorant statement I've ever heard. Please, people, for the love of Jesus, form a relationship, read your Bible and use what is taught in church to REALLY learn God's Word, not what RELIGION has taught you for 50 years. When I was in the world, dating women, drinking, smoking and doing whatever else your mind can think of, while the world and even some family would have sent me straight to hell that day if it was up to them, I am glad they don't have THAT POWER!

THERE IS A DIFFERENCE. Religion hinges on man-made rules and interpretations. By definition it is a set of deeply held personal or institutional beliefs or principles, according to Webster's dictionary.

Religion says if you ain't "living right," don't come to church.

Religion says a lot of things that someone has used from the Bible to create a rule based on their own interpretation. There is actually no Bible verse that says "come as you are." However, there are plenty of verses that speak on coming regardless of your sins, etc. Plus it has been taken completely out of context and used to relate to attire when it is not even talking about clothes.

Half the stuff people say ain't even in the Bible. Somebody said it in the pulpit and you have lived by it because you are too afraid to actually pick up your Bible except on Sunday morning. You can't promote the Word of God laced with condemnation and separation.

The one thing that made me so angry when I was in a relationship with a woman was that people would throw out Bible verses to condemn us but they never finished the verse. They always quoted 1 Corinthians 6:9 - 11 yet they only mentioned the sexually immoral part of the verse. I always took the chance to enlighten them that the same verse spoke of adulterers, idolaters, thieves, greed, drunkards and more. My simple stance was this: If you are going to bring me the Word, BRING IT ALL OUT. You can't throw out a part of a verse to condemn me on a certain lifestyle when the one you lead is also in the same verse next to mine.

If a Pastor takes issue with his member going somewhere else simply because they are seeking more than

Chapter 6

that house can give their spiritual growth or because they are not local anymore and need a covering, ask yourself, is his concern for my soul or my number on the roster?

I am so thankful Pastor Rodney Young taught me when I first left Newton to get under a covering wherever I went. He would say, "You know the Word so you will know if it is right." He even straightened me on my tithes and said, "You pay your tithes where you're getting fed. Sand Ridge will always be home but we want you under a good covering while you are away from home."

That, my friend, is a man of God.

Everything preached we should study ourselves to make sure WE know what it says and get an understanding. Some people cannot understand what they have never been exposed to. Preaching people happy is different from preaching and teaching people to peace and freedom. Being preached happy makes you feel awesome for a moment, while preaching and teaching people to peace and freedom arms us with what we need every day, not to be happy in the moment because it made us feel better. You feel better because you are growing in your own personal relationship and walk. So when the storm comes, you ain't got to call nobody to pray for you because you know it's already done for real for real.

My grandmother Johnnie Pearl said, "Getting baptized and not changing is like 'going down a dry devil and coming up a wet devil.'" Same devil!

November 26, 2019 – The day the shedding of fig leaves really took hold. My fig leaves were rooted in

what I had been taught about being a good girl so I could go to heaven: that I had to always do more, be more, push harder and reach higher. It was exhausting! My life was passing me by and I couldn't even remember the movie!

I remember reflecting on this day, thinking about the depression, secret therapy sessions, antidepressants I was taking and thinking, *You know what? I don't care if people know. I don't care if I am judged for taking care of my mental health. I don't care if people don't understand my journey.* I was no longer ashamed and seeking the approval of people through my accomplishments to drown the noise of my depression, pain and hurt. I didn't want them covered any longer. I wanted to heal.

November 27, 2019 – A day of removing fig leaves. The song "Deliver Me" got me right on through that. I listened to this song every day for weeks as I was praying for God to deliver me from my past pain. I don't mind worshipping in the car, in my office, in my room, while I clean, etc.

Remove that doubt! What else does God have to do? What is it that he has not done that would help you see how AWESOME HE IS?

I had to remove doubt that I would have the joy I saw others have in their walk. I had to learn the true joy is understanding that the Father loves me so much even when I have doubts, I still can have joy in knowing just who he is.

He alone is the keeper.

Chapter 6

- Moses doubted his ability because of his speech problem.
- Sarah doubted God's promise.
- Peter had doubts when walking on water.
- Gideon doubted being used singlehandedly against Israel's oppressors.

"The Devil cannot take what God has promised you but he can make it so hard you will surrender it yourself." – Bishop Joseph Walker III

I have always struggled with legalism in the body of Christ. I have always questioned why we do certain things under certain "denominations."

Listening to *Freedom from Legalism* by Dr. Tony Evans and reading Galatians 3!

"Legalism is seeking to relate to God by performance rather than relationship. It is a performance based relationship with God. The legalist says, 'I'm going to perform good so God likes me.'" – Dr. Tony Evans

My mom used to tell us, "If it ain't in that Bible or you can't read and understand it and what they are preaching is different, you get out of there."

Understand that obeying God's commandments is completely different than obeying manmade rules for "your" church. It is performance based vs. relational based.

"If you are serving Christ, coming to church, reading your Bible, praying and serving and all the other good religious stuff that you hear good Christians do—if you are doing those things out of Duty rather than Delight, your problem could be legalism." – Dr. Tony Evans

We should want to live in Christ because we love him; it should delight us to walk in his will. He loves us not because we are told we are going to hell if we don't do this and if we do that, not because we are told we MUST do this and that in order for him to love us.

He loves us regardless; whether we love him is the question.
John 8

Why would I go back to what God has brought me out of?

Chapter 7
Learning to walk

Boom! December 4, 2019 during a Women's Conference at the church, while Prophetess Deona Benson spoke, my spirit shifted and I BEGAN TO WALK without holding on to anything but the Word of God and his promise and purpose in and for my life. Right into Deliverance, Restoration, and Peace but best of all, Commitment to God and his purpose for my life. Let's not forget what I walked out of! Bondage, anger, depression, filling my life with food leading to obesity encompassed with physical illness, resentment and pure SIN.

December 9, 2019 – THE DAY I STARTED WALKING!

Stretcher turned Testimony Alert!

The enemy realized he couldn't get me through childhood trauma, unexpected death of my high school sweetheart and friend. His death almost took me out of here and no one even knew the suicide attempts. I finally got to the place of forgiveness and surrendering to God in 2018. The enemy figured out there was an anointing. ("Tell it right, baby" – Prophetess Deona Benson) on my life that wouldn't allow him to use that repeated childhood molestation and other trauma to keep a hold on me.

Here we are over a year later and I am ready to grow my hair back. I was in an appointed place at an appointed time for this very appointed reason.

I LAID IT DOWN SO I COULD LEVEL UP! I walked right into my anointing in this new decade. You can stay in CANNOT if you want to. I am taking up my stretcher and I am walking.

I was talking to my mama about that victory that morning and she said, "I know my part in it; back then, I was too drunk to raise y'all." I wanted to say, "Naw Mama it wasn't your fault," because IT WASN'T HER FAULT. But God said, "Let her own that place because a lot of people don't get parents like that. Let her speak that freedom to you. They don't get a parent who can say, 'Baby, I know it was bad but I can admit I didn't make it no better.'" My mama is FREE AND SAVED AND SO AM I.

My daddy, being a man of few words when he was mad, took care of it as any father would and never spoke a word about it. It was after his death that God revealed to me what my dad had done when he discovered what the person had done to me.

December 12, 2019 – The day I decided in order to go where God was taking me I had to get all the way in the Word of God. I didn't want to be like so many "saved" folks I knew who would whoop and holler in church and walk right out the doors to gossip. You

Chapter 7

know, the ones who are only saved on Sunday. That was not the kind of relationship I wanted. I wanted a genuine, honest and loving relationship with the Father.

Being sold into slavery didn't stop Joseph. Because of his gift from God, Joseph was able to interpret the dream of Pharaoh that others could not.

"Because it is necessary, now it is anointed." – Prophetess Deona Benson.

This gift enabled Joseph to rise to the point where he was able to give his father Jacob and brother's land in Rameses (the best of land in Egypt). The man (Pharaoh) instructed Joseph to give his father the land in Rameses (Genesis 47:5-6 and Genesis 47:11)—think about that for a moment.

"Baby, when it's your time, IT'S JUST YOUR TIME." – Prophetess Deona Benson

December 21, 2019 – The day I realized that in order to walk this thing out, I had to get up EVERY DAY SWINGING LIKE MY LIFE DEPENDED ON IT.

That time of the year is typically tough for me, not only because of the New Year date and sadness it brings me but also because I have to walk into another year, adding those we have lost in this year as well as years past. But I am going to celebrate all their lives this year! I am not going to lay in bed and cry the new-year in with pictures on the bed. I had lived in a world of severe depression all my life. The year 2012 knocked the wind out me with a death. In 2014, that whole year, from January 1–December 31 started a series of deaths so that each time I felt I got up, I was knocked back down. The whole time I just walked around working, going to school and raising kids. I cried myself to sleep almost every night of 2014, literally. I couldn't sleep at night without waking up crying. It was a dark place. This past decade has been a series of deaths, heartache and despair BUT BABY, I tell you I'm WALKING into 2020. When I tell people, "It's gonna be ok", it is because of the stretcher (like the man, I was carrying) and the ability to now carry the stretcher as a testimony!!!

I refused to stay there any longer because I realized grief is a process and I couldn't stay in the darkest place of it too long. I had to get up and WALK.

Psalms 73:26 NIV
My flesh and my heart may fail, but God is the strength of my heart and my portion forever.

Chapter 8
Whew, all this comes with being Saved?

The day I decided to refrain from sex until marriage, believe it or not, it had been a long while anyway, so why not? Moreover, it is the right thing to do. If I say I am saved, I don't want to be saved in one way and not in the other because I want to live in sin and be saved at the same time. That is a slippery slope to hell. Again, I wanted to do my walk the right way, not trying to be perfect but certainly to be intentional.

Let's talk taboo for one second. I get so sick of people saying, "It's just sex." My response now is, "It's just hell, and I don't like to burn."

Sex has really dominated the world of relationships. Don't let any man convince you to do anything you're not comfortable with. A man who cannot walk with you emotionally, spiritually and mentally, wait on your comfort level in certain areas like meeting kids, etc., to be ok and still love you, AIN'T THE ONE, SIS! Never compromise your beliefs rooted in the Word for any man.

When he says, "I love you and everything that comes with you. I'm going to go through whatever with you and for you. I am going to wait for whatever I have to because I want YOU"... and it didn't take having sex to get him to that place, SIS, he just may be the one! If by chance he is not then what have you lost? Not your integrity and abstinence. A lot of the heartache from dating comes from the disappointment and anger because we tend to compromise in ways we really didn't have to or need to then we are mad at ourselves in the end. I once told you I have three babies. Yeah, and I got them living in blatant sin. Know better, DO BETTER! Did I slip once or twice since January 2020? Yes, actually twice, but I repented and have since made a conscious effort not to put myself in a situation to be tempted. Now that is hard!

It was that day I decided I was no longer going to live with any kind of shame.

If a person is always focused on your past and who you USED to be and what you USED to do, you may have to WALK into your next phase and season letting their hand go. Be Unashamed, Be Bold in your changing in life. You can say whatever you want about who I used to be and what I used to do back then.

The reality is, you haven't known me since back then. I haven't been that person in many years anyway. My past doesn't shame me, baby! I carry my stretcher, honey.

It is the close of a DECADE. Don't walk into the next DECADE carrying the same baggage, in the same place mentally, emotionally and spiritually.

Chapter 9
Leaving the Broken, Bitter Girl in the Last Decade

It was only the second day in the new decade and the enemy was trying his best to consume my mind and heart with grief. I would have a moment here and there but I refused to stay there and wallow in it. I was told to do something and I was fighting against it. Not because I didn't want to but because I was letting other people's mistakes create doubt in my mind. I listened to a video yesterday and I have listened to it several times. Jameliah Gooden aid, "God will hurt your feelings to save you" as she spoke on Paul's deliverance. It was on my mind this morning to listen to it again. She was discussing Paul!!!

I like studying Paul. His journey amazes me. In reading it this morning (Acts 9) the part that seemed to jump out at me was his loss of sight for three days after he began his journey as Paul. Ananias was sent to lay hands on him, restoring his sight. He tried to reason with God by only seeing all the bad done but he went and Paul's sight was restored. Ananias was STUCK in Saul's mistakes. God had to let him know what he saw had nothing to do with what God was seeing for Paul's future. It always amazed me that in changing Saul's life, his name changed to.

I thank God I am a new creature! I don't associate with that little broken girl, that bitter, angry woman anymore. Sometimes people associate our past with the new creature and they try to reason with God when he is calling them to do something in our lives. Get out of my mistakes and bring me what God has told you to; I am waiting! Stop looking back at the past and mistakes of others and do what God has told you to do. I am your Ananias; get ready because I am coming and I bring light and sight with me, whether you want it or not. I'm doing what I am told to do regardless of how I feel in the flesh about it. If my spirit is moved to do it, I'M COMING!! What you do with it is on you.

Chapter 10
Freedom from Church Hurt

It is tough when you've been "church hurt"—been there, done that, got the t-shirt!

We lose sight that it is not the "church" that is the issue but people in the church. I started looking at it like this: It is no different than the people at our jobs and even in some of our families; that is the same way the "church folk" are. I had to learn that not going to church didn't hurt anybody but me. The building didn't hurt me, people did, so I had to refocus my mindset before I took myself to hell.

As I listened to New Year, New You pt. 2 by Pastor Gregg Magee Sr., reading Acts 21, I am always amazed how Peter stood at the door knocking and those praying for him thought Rhonda was going crazy.

The very man they were praying for God had brought him out and there he stood. While they stood amazed, Peter was calm as he gave them instructions, then he was out. Don't worry about those people in the church looking at you when you show up, just go on. Like Peter, stay calm and know God brought you out so you're going there is not for the people, it is for you! Out of all those people considered "fake Christians," all we need is one real one to help us through the door. As Pastor Gregg Magee says, "ONE person is ineffective, but give me another person who is gonna touch and agree in the spirit of God, and baby, we're onto something."

Hebrews 10:25, NIV
Let us not give up meeting together, as some are in the habit of doing, but let us encourage one another—and all the more as you see the Day approaching.

Church is not to "Save" us. Our relationship with God does that part.

Church is not to go "not be depressed." Unless you surrender and allow God to move, we are back at square one by the evening. Church is a place for us to go be among people who have been where we are. To get under the leadership of a good shepherd to help us in our personal walk and a church family that is going to love us and hold us accountable.

A person can go to church every day and still die and go to hell. What do you go to church for?

The pastor preached on the prophet Elijah. As he ran down the line of things God had done pertaining to Elijah as he sat in isolation in such a depressed state, it reminded me of how we often FORGET where God has brought us from in times past. I am guilty of being in a place where God had to remind me just how far he has brought me. We cry and remind God of the dark places we are in, forgetting all about the dark places he has brought us out of. As he spoke on that topic, I was internally grieved as even in my spiritual growth, I have to constantly remind myself where God has brought me from. I felt guilty for having to remind myself so much then I realized, at least I am reminding myself to keep me WALKING!

Chapter 11

How hard is Godly Discipline?

I will answer that for you: VERY HARD sometimes. During this time, I learned what it really meant for the flesh to have to die daily. Now, every time I am at such a point I recall Paul asking God to remove the thorn and God reminding him his Grace is sufficient. I sometimes must remind myself I am not that person anymore so I can get back in alignment. Oh, she is still in there and sometimes it is tough to keep her at bay. I have some things I feel I need more discipline in before God is able to move me to the next place in those particular seasons. Thank God simply for being able to understand those areas in which I wrestle so I won't forget.

Many times we "blame God" for our hardships and storms when half of the time we went against what God was telling us in the first place.

Proverbs 12:1 (LEB) – He who loves discipline loves knowledge, but he who hates rebuke is stupid.

Personal Discipline and Stewardship have been two of my biggest struggles personally. Working out consistently is my first step in discipline. It requires no one really counting on me except those who cheer me on in the journey. If I don't go, it is really my choice BUT I want to share my journey with integrity so I get up not only for me but for someone else to say I can do that. However, because I know my journey will help someone on their journey, even on the days I feel like I don't want to fight, work out, study, pray or whatever, I ask God to kill the flesh and guide me. It usually turns out to be just what I needed at the moment.

Chapter 12
The day I decided to stop robbing God!

In reflection over my life I noticed God has truly significantly blessed me in various areas of my life. Then there are areas in my life where I say, "Lord, when is this gonna change?" The pastor preached on Stewardship as a matter of the Heart. I understood and I have been mindful ever since, YET I still have areas where I am continuously working on my stewardship.

My one Goal for 2020 was to be a 10% tither and to improve my Financial and Parental Stewardship—simple as that. Let me tell you all something, until I got it down in my heart for real, I still struggled with tithing. Every now and then, I still have a brief thought when I prepare to tithe that diverts to bills and what all I have to pay. Sometimes I have to talk to myself or the enemy and say NO I am not robbing the God I serve. I try to make sure I tithe before I do anything else with any increase I receive to help me stay on track.

Keep me and my tithing in prayer constantly, you hear me?

Luke 16:10, KJV – He that is faithful in that which is least is faithful also in much: and he that is unjust in the least is unjust also in much.

Luke 16 is a parable told by Jesus of a steward who was dishonest and mismanaging. His stewardship was taken away.

"With Freedom comes responsibility." – Dr. Tony Evans

I have always disliked when people do not take responsibility for their actions. It burns me up! Blame covers responsibility in my eyes. I speak about Integrity to my kids ALL the time.

"Deliverance is not the same as Freedom. Deliverance gains you the opportunity to pursue freedom." – Dr. Tony Evans

As the year has rolled on, I have found myself making sure to tithe, not because I am afraid of what others thought but because I truly believe in the principle and in being faithful to God in all areas. Even if I slip every now and then, the wonderful thing about him is he still loves me. I can't blame the food for my years of obesity! I chose to eat badly, I chose not to care. I can't blame my finances on not being a faithful tither in the past because I have the free will to choose to or not to.

Many people struggle with the principle of tithing. The negative commentary from people misusing the Bible for greed has warped society's mindset on tithing in the spiritual sense of sowing. The Bible speaks several times about people not being obedient. The principle of tithing is a heart thing, as Pastor Gregg Magee taught it. The mindset shouldn't be, "Let me go on and give them this money before they start talking about paying tithes;" that is not cheerful giving. You just keep it and go on about your business. If your heart ain't right then why even do it?

The mindset should be, "Lord, I love you and I want to abide by what Your Word says."

Malachi 3:6–9, KJV – For I am the Lord, I change not; Therefore, ye sons of Jacob are not consumed. Even from the days of your fathers ye are gone away from mine ordinances, and have not kept them. Will a man rob God? Yet ye have robbed me. But ye say, Wherein have we robbed thee? In tithes and offerings. Ye are cursed with a curse: for ye have robbed me, even this whole nation.

We should ask ourselves how we can follow all the other principles and commandments, yet this ONE many of us have failed to follow. We say we love God, yet we would still ROB him. I don't know about you, but I sure wouldn't rob a person on this side of heaven. I try to make sure now that I keep this one fact at the forefront of my mind. Even deeper than this is the fact that tithing has been taught so harshly over the years that we have failed to understand it truly is a matter of the heart, as Pastor Gregg Magee Sr. preached once before. While I wasn't necessarily convicted by the message at the time, it gave me a deeper understanding of tithing, far beyond "just giving money to the church."

Malachi 3:10-12, KJV – Bring ye all the tithes into the storehouse, that there may be meat in mine house, and prove me now herewith, saith the Lord of hosts, if I will not open you the windows of heaven, and pour you out a blessing, that there shall not be room enough to receive it. And I will rebuke the devourer for your sakes, and he shall not destroy the fruits of your ground; neither shall your vine cast her fruit before the time in the field, saith the Lord of hosts.

And all nations shall call you blessed: for you shall be a delightsome land, saith the Lord of hosts.

Look, for a while on payday as God was working on me with tithing, I would have to repeat these words to myself so I wouldn't try to talk myself out of paying my tithes: "Lord crucify this flesh and rise up in me." No, for real, this was my simple prayer on payday, when my check hit the bank, to help me stay on track with keeping my tithing first.

1 Samuel 15:22, KJV – And Samuel said, Hath the LORD as great delight in burnt offerings and sacrifices, as in obeying the voice of the LORD? Behold, to obey is better than sacrifice, and to hearken than the fat of rams.

Stop letting people around you influence your obedience. Get in the Word for yourself and let God work on YOUR HEART. I stand on the tithing principal because I have done it and continue to do it and IT WORKS. Every word in the Word of God rings true in all areas so certainly tithing does as well, my friend.

Chapter 13
Lord, I just got off the Walker; how am I going to show someone how to use it?

When the shift really started to happen—when I began to Walk!

Hey, you see her? She has known her calling for many years. She shied away from people, alienating herself because it was hard for her to deal with people and the Word of God not spill from her mouth. She kept saying, "Lord, not yet; Lord, it is not the right time," BUT in March 2019 after being beaten, broken and bound she walked into a PLACE where she said, "Lord, I am ready but my feet won't move." She began to feel a change in her spirit, that gift of ministering to people that others had spoken to her. She would be in a dark place herself and people would call her or come see her and God would manifest a Word from her lips, then when they would leave she would ask, "Now Lord, where did that come from?"

I can't tell you how many times over the last five years I was asked, "Are you a minister?" and I would reply, "Naw man, I just love God and I know what you're going through." I grew up singing in the choir with a voice that could have been used to knock the congregation off their feet. My aunt used to get so mad because I wouldn't sing in that place because I knew while it was one of my talents, it was not my Gift. I wrestled with depression, past failures and emotional bondage but I always knew there was a way out. I walked into The Empowerment Ministries Christian Center (EMCC) saying, "Lord, I know what I am supposed to be doing but my feet won't move." God began to peel back the layers and fig leaves that were keeping my feet from moving to get me to December 5, 2019, when he said to me "It is time to WALK".

That "wise beyond my years" wisdom that you see is not me. It is the calling. That being able to hold it together during death literally ushering in God while watching several people close to me take their last breath, that strength the world sees, IS THAT CALLING. On June 25, 2019, I lay beside my daddy and ministered to him on his way to gain his wings, telling him how grateful we were to have him and what a wonderful father he was. When he gained those wings the HUMAN IN ME wanted to scream and cry but that SPIRITUAL PLACE only allowed me to cry out, "THANK YOU, GOD." Everyone around at that moment couldn't understand what I was thanking God for when my daddy just gained his wings. I thanked him the suffering didn't last long. I thanked him for the years we had. I thanked him that he made provision for my daddy to rededicate his life before he gave him rest.

See the human is hurt, the spirit rejoices.

Chapter 13

I didn't say I was a pastor; I didn't say I was trying to get in a pulpit. WHAT I SAID WAS I AM NOW WALKING INTO ACCEPTING THE LOVING ON PEOPLE AND SPEAKING INTO THEIR SITUATION THROUGH GENERAL CONVERSATION MINISTERING, A CALLING THAT HAS BEEN ON MY LIFE SINCE I WAS YOUNG AND I AM UNASHAMED OF IT! As I sat there that night saying, "I got it" to the Lord the song "It's important to me that I'm saved" started playing in my head.

When I began to understand how my gift of Leadership is also a Gift for the Ministry.

It has always been important to me to be a good leader to those God blesses me to lead. I have served in leadership since the age of 25, to many who are older than me. God blessed me with an empathetic spirit of leadership that exceeds anything I could have ever imagined. Leadership and Ministry of any kind is service to others. It requires an unimaginable sacrifice mentally and emotionally to help those we lead both professionally and personally. It is continuous learning, as none of us truly arrive because none of us are perfect.

The willingness and gift of leadership hinges on understanding the needs of our teams over our own desires. A true leader is always coachable, open, assertive, and humble, values their team and their separate strengths, accountable and holds themselves to a higher sense of integrity and character than anyone else ever could. They ensure their team understands they will get right in the trenches with them.

A true leader is not about the front but ensuring we all move safely and effectively while making a difference

TOGETHER. That was the moment God started peeling back the layers of legalism and religion to reveal Freedom and Love.

Ok Lord, I hear you.

Then my mind asked, "Lord, you told Jeremiah that You knew him before you formed him in his mother's belly; why allow Saul to do all the destruction he did?" Immediately, I heard, "In order to get where I'm taking you, I have to allow the free will of man and the choices therein but when it is time and you have not stepped into what I have laid out for you, I WILL KNOCK YOU DOWN TO STAND YOU UP!"

The enemy didn't knock Paul off the horse, GOD DID! The devil didn't blind Him, GOD DID. (I actually said, "Help me, Holy Ghost" in my head after that part).

Sometimes the mess we are in is because we are not listening to God. We just keep galloping until GOD has to knock us down and blind us so we can't see the path backwards until we can see it as the PAST.

HEY YOU—yeah, you—no, *us* saved folk, don't be like Ananias unless you are already on your way to do what God has told you to do. Stop looking at folk and trying to reason with God on why you shouldn't do what he told you to do in their life.

Somebody is walking around here blind because you want to be hardheaded.

Go give those folks their sight!!

Chapter 13

February 8, 2020 – The day I realized I was involuntarily morphing right into what God called me to be. As I sat in front of the promotion board that morning, not a nerve was rattled. I answered questions as if I was speaking to a crowd. As I sat and waited to see the Wing Commander and Command Chief, what I thought would be a quick five minutes of congratulations turned into a full-fledged conversation on how inspiring my story is and how proud they were of me.

In that very moment is when I heard God say, "These are the moments the storms were for. This is why I kept whispering to you through the trials."

July 29, 2020 – The day I became a published author and realized how my testimony will help someone.

As I received the flyer for *The Mom in Me* anthology, I realized my prayer for God to help me become a better mother was happening as the chapter "Mommy is Depressed" forced me into dark places that I hated. Places I never wanted to see again. Having to face them, it was easy for me to say those words to my children and apologize to them for any effects my severe depression had on them during that dark time. It was freeing, to say the least. Also during this time, I was engaged in a Small Group on Spiritual Warfare and learning how to really armor up for the daily battle, even though I already knew who had the victory. This was the exact moment when I realized my testimonies in life were for something bigger than me and I needed to share them with others so they know IT IS ONLY A VALLEY AND NOT OUR DESTINATION!

Chapter 14
The journey continues; PRESS FORWARD

August 13, 2020 – The day it sank in Regardless of whether I have to journey alone, it is a journey worth taking.

As I took part in a Zoom session and the leader spoke, certain things were confirmation on some areas of prayer. Then she said something which resonated with my spirit so profoundly that all I could do was thank God for the Word. It was that intense. See, when we become saved, when we REALLY become saved and WANT to love God, treat people right and love on people, honor God and be steadfast and immovable, the enemy sends areas where we doubt. For me, in that time, it was this very testimonial book. It wasn't that I cared about being so transparent. My concern was related to whether it would do what it is purposed to do: help free people, help someone know the battle is already won and to just stay the course. However, there was a brief moment before the Zoom session where I said, "What, people don't understand the why?" As she spoke, she used the very words God spoke to me hours before: "This is only a portion." Prophetess Deona Benson went on to say later on in the session, "Your journey cannot be based on how many people understand and agree! You cannot delay based on others' inability to understand or refusal to support it."

While she was not in that moment speaking directly to me, the spirit was... GOD WAS.

Afterword

May this shared journey not only remind you of the love of Christ but also that in his love for us, we already have the Victory. There really is no war to win, as it has already been won.

There are times we have to endure the Valley on the road to our Victory.

So as this year continues to roll on, make no mistake, deliverance and freedom are NOT a one-time deal. It is a daily journey in life and the daily walk—constant "Word, Worship and Warfare," according to Pastor Gregg Magee Sr. It is a conscious process of being able to divide my flesh from my spiritual man. Do I always get it right? Heck no, but I try to always go back to what I know to be right and acknowledge when my flesh has gotten the best of me. I am excited about what God has in store not only for me but for you as well.

The journey continues, a valley here, a victory there. The difference now is that instead of despair, I see victory. Even if I have to see it through tears, I know it is there. Death anniversaries and other life stressors, and then, as if that wasn't enough, we are in the middle of a pandemic—yet press forward!

AJ Riley

www.ingramcontent.com/pod-product-compliance
Lightning Source LLC
Chambersburg PA
CBHW072016060426
42446CB00043B/2566